# Table of Contents

Advanced Sleep Phase Disorder: Causes, Symptoms, and Treatment Options

# Advanced Sleep Phase Disorder: Symptoms, Causes, and Treatment

# 1. Introduction to Advanced Sleep Phase Disorder

This text is focused on offering an in-depth understanding of advanced sleep phase disorder and is divided into three sections. Following this introduction, one section will be on understanding advanced sleep phase disorder symptoms. This section will delve deeply into concepts like symptoms of advanced sleep phase disorder, insomnia, causes of advanced sleep phase disorder, mental health, mood, external factors and signs, depression, and treatment options that include recent advances in treatment. The next section is focused on understanding advanced sleep phase disorder causes. The section is set to provide a comprehensive and detailed understanding of causes that include mental health and medical history or physical conditions. The last section involves treating advanced sleep phase disorder. We look at the importance of sleep, types of treatment, advanced sleep phase disorder for changing external environmental cues, and other treatments offered for miserable sleep. Finally, the section will also offer an up-to-date look at several drugs that have shown some promise when it comes to treating advanced sleep phase disorder.

Today, modern psychiatry and psychology systems offer thorough insight into sleep disorders that often occur as a result of mental or emotional stress. Advanced sleep phase disorder is one such disorder that results from poor mental health and medical history. Advanced sleep phase disorder can be extremely harmful as this disorder can affect an individual's mental health and sometimes cause depression. Besides, this disorder's symptoms can cause other sleep disorders and may often lead to uneasiness.

## 2. Understanding Sleep and Circadian Rhythms

Circadian disorders are disturbances of the rhythm. A person's normal wake-up time is shifted earlier. Individuals mostly feel sleepy in the early evening and that progressively changes if allowed to move to an earlier bedtime. Circadian rhythm disorders in individuals are linked with reduced sleep quality and functioning. Advanced sleep phase disorder is one of them. The disorder related changes in a person's dinner time and sign of sleep that increase in the afternoon and decreases in the morning. The person mostly sleeps between 7-9 pm in the evening and frequently wakes around 2-3 am.

Sleep is a condition of the body and mind which typically recurs for several hours every night, in which the nervous system is relatively inactive, the postural muscles relaxed, and consciousness practically suspended. This is contrasted with wakefulness, in which our body cycles through alert states of higher mental function. Within a 24-hour day, numerous patterns are exhibited by the body, with hormonal release, regulation of blood pressure, body temperature, and many other activities being performed daily. These patterns are known as circadian rhythms and are managed by the light and dark cycles of the environment and cues from behaviors and meals. The interplay of circadian rhythms and sleep has a broad impact on performance, mood, and overall health of individuals. Sleep is controlled by the homeostatic drive-sleep pressure that increases the longer the person is awake. This drive is also regulated by their circadian rhythm and time of day. Sleep patterns and circadian rhythms differ with genetic and age too.

## 2.1. The Importance of Sleep

Sleep Disorders: The main purpose of treatment therapies and surveys is to get an insight into and to assess sleep disorders. Sleep disorders are not necessarily diseases. Any alterations in healthy sleep-wake parameters are responsible for either the association of the disorder or the disease. Sleep disorders have the potential to interrupt normal sleep-wake cycles by affecting the sleep duration and believed to be immediately created or induced.

The purpose of sleep is still unknown, but it is stated as the final recovery of the body. Healthy sleep is vital for our overall health, well-being, and mental functioning. Sleep loss or deprivation impinges adversely on physical health by impacting the immune system which raises the possibility of infections. Healthy sleep-wake patterns are crucial for cognitive functions and managing emotions. Furthermore, good sleep-wake cycles prepare individuals for next intellectual tasks and physical activities. Good sleep-wake patterns directly impact the cardiovascular system of a human's body by lowering the glucose levels in an individual's body, thus preventing an individual from diabetes. Successive treatment therapies are designed to improve sleep-wake patterns as irregular patterns are responsible for certain disorders such as mental illness, mood disorders, and anxiety.

Inadequate sleep impacts more on younger adults, who have to raise their children and maintain households due to which they go through very little sleep.

The sleep-wake cycle is vital for various functions of the human body. A good sleep-wake cycle is essential for maintaining good mental and physical well-being. Sleep hygiene is important, which is a practice for the improvement of sleep. For a good sleep-wake cycle, sleep latency (time taken by an individual to fall asleep) is crucial, and it directly affects...

## 2.2. The Role of Circadian Rhythms

The process of falling and staying asleep is also partially controlled by a specialized mechanism in the brain that regulates our drive to stay awake called the sleep-wake homeostasis. Besides feeling very tired after having pushed through many nights with little sleep, we can also interpret the strength of this drive when we are able to sleep without interruptions. The interplay of these rhythms and wakefulness and sleep help to maintain a delicate balance in which we move through sleep cycles throughout the night. When interrupted, this can cause us to feel groggy and unfocused during the day. Given that some individuals possess circadian rhythms that result in feeling sleepy earlier than the average person, or being ready to rise and shine before the sun comes up, it's understandable that the right circumstances may lead to developing a condition like advanced sleep phase disorder.

Your circadian rhythms are an integral part of your biological makeup, governing your physical, mental, and behavioral changes throughout a 24-hour cycle. They influence a litany of bodily functions and processes, including, but not limited to, hormone production, blood pressure, and body temperature. Each person's circadian rhythms can differ somewhat depending on certain factors like genetics and age. When kept in good working order, your circadian rhythms make it intuitive to understand when it's time to go to bed and when you should be waking up. One key element of our circadian rhythms is sleep. Our awake-sleep schedules are dictated by the natural cycles of light and darkness, which help to signal to our body when it's time to wind down and when it's time to rise and shine. Such signals help in part to illustrate why our circadian rhythms inform when we feel most sleepy.

# 3. Types of Sleep Disorders

Sleep apnea is a dangerous medical condition that causes a person to stop breathing up to hundreds of times per night. It can cause stress on the heart, reducing its efficiency in doing its job. Advanced sleep phase disorder is a condition also known as familial advanced sleep phase syndrome (FASPS), which arises when an individual's internal sleep-wake clock advances at least two hours before the clock of typical older adults. It develops a reduced duration of the relative nocturnal sleep period and frequent symptoms during the evening as a result of chronic phase advance. This low-prevalence disorder shows variable symptoms, severity, age at onset, and human circadian period across families with autosomal dominant inheritance. Families have allowed multisystem research to explore the biology underlying circadian phase and determine the contribution of circadian disruption to mood and neurologic disorders.

Sleep disorders can affect different people in different ways. Some can be damaging and make it difficult to live, while others can be mild, which can still lower the quality of life. It can cause significant health problems and impair a significant amount of motor skills and cognitive functions. Sleep disorders could include insomnia, sleep apnea, advanced sleep phase disorder, and many more. Insomnia is a condition where one can't sleep, can't stay asleep, or has poor underlying sleep patterns, which results in mental and physical distress.

## 3.1. Overview of Sleep Disorders

Parasomnias cover a diverse group of disorders involving unwanted events that interfere with sleep. Several of these events including REM sleep behavior disorder, sleep paralysis, night terrors, sleepwalking, sleep talking, nocturnal leg cramps, bruxism, sleep enuresis, and teeth grinding are recognized as separate disorders in their own right, based on their presentation. Lastly, sleep-related movements include restless leg syndrome (RLS) and periodic limb movement disorder (PLMD). The circadian rhythm sleep disorders are a family of disorders in which the timing of sleep is constitutionally or environmentally out of alignment. Giving delayed sleep phase disorder as an example, these conditions can result (as with advanced sleep phase disorder) from endogenous factors, environmental factors, or a mix of both.

Sleep disorders encompass a broad spectrum of conditions that impact the initiation and maintenance of sleep, the timing and regularity of sleep schedule, and the resulting experience of wakefulness and daytime functioning. Disorders of initiating and maintaining sleep are essentially the insomnias and generally relate to a person's ability to fall asleep (termed sleep onset) and/or to stay asleep through the night (termed sleep maintenance). Sleep insufficiency, or the inability to sleep an adequate amount, can be chronic or situationally related. Hypersomnia encompasses a large group of disorders and refers to excess sleepiness or excessive time spent asleep.

It can refer to disorders with long sleeping hours or normal sleeping hours.

## 3.2. Classification of Sleep Disorders

The following classification attempts are also based on dyssomnias. This issue has not entered any classification based on the criteria of causing or not causing clinical suffering, but it is interesting to point out that a sleep disorder that does not generate more impairment, in addition to the possibility of being considered healthy or sick, is taken as a pathological condition requiring treatment. In these latest classifications, we are charged with analyzing a chronic sleep disorder that causes significant distress, persists for a period of time, and causes marked impairment in personal, social, occupational, or academic functioning. Some of those sleep disorders are considered limited in duration, while others last as long as the conditions.

Leaving aside the classification of lupus, fatigue, or exhaustion, sleep problems are usually divided into parasomnias and dyssomnias. Parasomnias include unwanted physical events, sensations, and actions when the person is asleep or when she is transitioning between the various waking and sleeping states. As an example, we can include the well-known nightmare, which is a complex sleep disorder. The so-called Nightmare Disorder or Nightmare Disorder appears in the International Classification of Sleep Disorders and the DSM-5, and it is usually diagnosed using the clinical criteria that disappear in both charts. The Sleep-Wake Disorders of the DSM-5 also includes a category for the Nightmare Disorder, with the essential feature of recurrent awakenings with recall of intensely disturbing dreams usually involving fear.

# 4. Advanced Sleep Phase Disorder: Definition and Overview

It can occur either due to intrinsic factors, which are related to an in-built proclivity. This could be the case when the disorder starts at a very young age for a patient. Heredity seems also to play a role, as it is common for patients with ASPD to have relatives that also have the disorder. Delayed sleep phase syndrome, which is closely related to ASPD, is the opposite of ASPD, meaning patients go to bed rather late. This syndrome also runs in families, and in some cases, the syndrome can shift from a delayed to an advanced phase according to the time of life of the patient. This helps to prove the common underlying cause for the disorders. Acquired advanced sleep phase disorder is when brain injuries occur, having a physical impact on the sleep-wake center in the brain is also a possible cause for this disorder. Syndromes like ASPD usually describe a form of a particular disorder which can occur as a primary or as a secondary occurrence.

Advanced sleep phase disorder (ASPD) is a circadian rhythm sleep disorder characterized by a consistency within the patient regarding their complaints. The main problem with ASPD is the fact that even though patients can sleep rather easily, they tend to wake up very early in the morning, usually around 3:00 a.m. to 5:00 a.m. This is consistently the case, even on days when these individuals are allowed to sleep in longer, and it's happening against the patient's will. The adverse effects of waking up with the birds are the main reason patients seek help.

Advanced Sleep Phase Disorder – Definition and Overview

## 4.1. Characteristics of Advanced Sleep Phase Disorder

ASPD was originally conceived of as a disorder that primarily affected older adults, many of whom were institutionalized or retired at the time of discovery. Although it is considered a clinically rare disorder, a small number of general population studies have provided an assessment of ASPD prevalence. ASPD is characterized as having a high familial aggregation, which suggests a genetic predisposition. While it is commonly referred to as a type of CRSD, it has also been suggested to be a type of sleep disorder budding off from the other CRSDs as well. Even though ASPD can occur at any age, it more often occurs in older adults who have an earlier than usual need to sleep and wake up. Unlike delayed sleep phase disorder and non-24-hour sleep-wake rhythm disorder, which typically appear during adolescence or early adulthood, ASPD usually appears after the age of 30.

Advanced sleep phase disorder (ASPD) is a circadian rhythm sleep disorder (CRSD) that is characterized by a chronotype-related shift of sleep start and stop times earlier than what is considered normal. Most CRSDs exhibit bothersome symptoms such as insomnia, excessive daytime sleepiness, or irregular sleep-wake patterns. ASPD, however, is distinct from other CRSDs because it is primarily considered a disorder of timing. There are no known unique symptoms associated with ASPD that do not also occur concomitantly with other CRSDs. Its main manifestation is related to the mistiming of its two cardinal symptoms: delayed sleep onset and wake-up time.

# 5. Symptoms of Advanced Sleep Phase Disorder

Primary symptoms of advanced sleep phase disorder include being unable to fall asleep, being unable to stay asleep, waking up too early, and excessive sleepiness during the day. Secondary symptoms of advanced sleep phase disorder that might be related to being unable to fall asleep include tardiness, school or life time work absenteeism, uncontrollable crying, and disguising exploitation such as theft, as these patients yearn to partly compensate or catch up on lost sleep at bedtime with sleep studyless qualification. Excessive sleepiness can be related to being unable to stay asleep, as a limited total sleeping time in the night causes the body shift more sleepiness to the day in an automatic compensation mechanism.

Because symptoms of advanced sleep phase disorder in children and adults differ, a child may be misdiagnosed with attention deficit hyperactivity disorder (ADHD). This is especially true for females who have an ADHD diagnosis. Symptoms primarily correspond to when a person goes to sleep and awakes. They include difficulties with the amount of sleep, falling asleep, staying asleep, behaviors in sleep, fatigue, or feeling unrefreshed. Symptoms can occur on a continuum from mild to severe. Advanced sleep phase symptoms can either be primary or secondary.

## 5.1. Primary Symptoms

It is important to rule out comprehensive napping and perhaps an insufficient total sleep time as a cause of the early bedtime. In our clinical program years ago, we noted that when patients were instructed to refrain from nap taking, the time of seeking their beds would fall back closer to the typical range of bedtimes during the week. Also, we've also noted that using actigraphy recording, people (adult males and the elderly in particular) who have advanced bedtimes had a relatively early rise time, which if coupled with a short bedtime could bring about what appears to be chronic sleep deprivation.

People with advanced sleep phase disorder typically present with a period of several hours every evening during which they feel very sleepy and usually go to bed quite early. This is in contrast to the better-known problem of wanting to sleep for a period of hours later than a person desires, such as cannot fall asleep before midnight or does not wish to wake up in the morning before 10 am. In the general public, this latter problem is often not seen as a very unusual complaint, but people who come in seeking help usually indicate that they have struggled with delayed sleep-wake patterns for many years. Generally, no other major sleep or psychiatric disorder is found to cause or maintain the advanced sleep phase problem. While as many as 40% of patients report a family history of advancing circadian patterns; about one third have a first or second-degree relative with the same advanced sleep phase schedule. Perhaps because this is one of the rarest of all sleep disorders, males and females seem equally affected. The diagnosis of advanced sleep phase disorder is confirmed by decreasing phase angle on the DLMO, or sleep atop the core body temperature minimum.

## 5.2. Secondary Symptoms

To be certain of a diagnosis of advanced sleep phase disorder, one must suffer from symptoms for at least 3 months. Commonly, patients have multiple stages of sleep need that are unsatisfied for years without encountering symptoms in childhood or adolescence. The quantity of sleep necessary to match personal demands changes throughout life; it is typical to need more rest in adolescence. It is difficult to analyze the initial time at which issues arise if symptoms were not severe when the patient is examined. Family histories of early wakers or parents with DSPS are commonly seen in patients. Extreme chronotypes, such as severe DSPS and ASPD, are more common in close relatives of DSPS individuals than in the total population.

It is notable that advanced sleep phase disorder, when not interfering with social or occupational schedules, is often an asymptomatic condition. Nevertheless, its main symptoms, getting sleepy and waking up early, may lead to different manifestations as a secondary consequence of broken sleep patterns. Waking up numerous times throughout the evening can result in sleep fragmentation or "non-restful sleep," which has potential as a secondary inducer of daytime tiredness. However, it appears as if most patients reach their possible sleep schedule, at which point it is challenging to become more tired. The most frequent secondary issue is the development of anxiety, despair, and impairments in public and workplace functioning. The Ullanlinna Narcolepsy Scale and the

Epworth Sleepiness Scale can frequently reveal concerns of
weariness.

# 6. Causes and Risk Factors

The circadian rhythm is heavily influenced by genetic factors, as is almost anything else in the body, and that is most likely why advanced sleep phase disorder can run in families. Scientists have identified a few mutations in specific genes that are associated with the rare forms of advanced sleep phase disorder. One gene in particular, PER2, has been shown to play an important role in maintaining the circadian rhythm in the human body. There may be other genes playing a role in advanced sleep phase disorder, but these have not yet been discovered. It is not known whether the PER2 mutation is already present when a baby is born or if it is acquired at some point in early development. It is not known how, when, or why the PER2 gene might mutate. It is also not known if the disease can manifest either with or without the gene expression.

Risk factors Your risk of developing advanced sleep phase disorder may increase if you: • Are a 65-year-old adult or older • Have a family history of advanced sleep phase disorder

• Advanced sleep phase disorder can be caused or exacerbated by mutations in certain genes or, less frequently, by other underlying medical, neurological, or sleep disorders. • In most cases, the cause of advanced sleep phase disorder is not known and it is not related to any other condition. • Though the exact prevalence of advanced sleep phase disorder is not currently known, some evidence suggests that more than 1 in 300 adults suffers from the condition, and it is more prevalent in older adults than in younger individuals.

What are the causes and risk factors for advanced sleep phase disorder?

## 6.1. Biological Factors

Moreover, given that circadian light sensitivity has been demonstrated to be relatively preserved in these individuals, ASWD might be more indicative of increased non-photic factors contributing to chronotype than the actual manifestation of symptoms, which are likely to be exacerbated by age-related reductions in neurotensin and orexin. This possible involvement of the non-photic factors in ASWD pathophysiology has potential implications for treatment, as it would ultimately suggest that the development of type-specific management strategies for evening chronotypes may not be the most appropriate approach to the treatment of ASWD. Moreover, if someone with a SSN T6 was to wake up at 5:30, their threshold for light-induced phase-shifting might potentially be half or below threshold.

The process of habitual bed and rise times can have profound health and wellbeing implications beyond what happens to align with an individual's innate circadian tendency. Occurring more often in elderly adults, various factors have been implicated in the development and perpetuation of ASWD, including alterations in the melatonin threshold and increases in hyperarousal. Unlike evening chronotypes, for whom the symptoms of delayed sleep phase disorder are typically a result of social and environmental factors, advanced sleep times seem to be more driven by internal biological processes. Of relevance to this are reports of ASWD symptoms in blind individuals without light perception. Although there is much to be learnt about the factors contributing to ASWD in this population, the circadian oscillator has been demonstrated to be capable of maintaining such intrinsic periods in isolation, although it is done so with an altered relationship with clock time, which is often longer than 24h.

## 6.2. Genetic Factors

Despite the suspected high dominance of the underlying genes, the clinical syndrome might occur sporadically in some people. This hereditary property of the advanced sleep phase disorder also helps illuminate the unusual findings on depression and mental disease. Thus, a preexistent vulnerability has another genetically linked disease with irregular depression onset, which can be the antecedent or associative issue following the decade's long diurnal sleep rhythm.

It is also known that the genetic factors linked to advanced sleep phase disorder include occurrences in close and extended families. Family history studies show that one individual in the family frequently has one or both parents with an earlier sleep onset and offset. Thus, it is suggested that the initial development of the sleep timing characteristic of advanced sleep phase disorder people is in part hereditary. At least three genetic factors influence the advancedness of the sleep-wake cycles. The first is a variant in the gene period 3, which has a small effect but is quite easy to assess. This mutation causes the encoded protein to be made into a double portion and degrade faster. The mutation makes the endogenous rhythm period ($\tau$) time shorter; the gene that carries the mutation time duration is consequently advanced. The overall percentage of cases is quite different among advanced sleep phase disorder compared to married persons with no history of such sleep disorder. 39 percent have extended family members with advanced sleep phase disorder, while only 2 percent of spouses are detected with advanced sleep phase disorder. In summary, results supporting a chronic hereditary basis suggest an autosomal dominant inheritance model for the extreme advancedness of the sleep-wake phase of patients with advanced sleep phase disorder. The high percentage of affected individuals over the lifetime of any persons in the family suggests that disease root genes, unless completely penetrable, are of high dominance.

Alone or together with endogenous sleep disorders, advanced sleep phase disorders can be treated several ways. Three well-established treatment methods for circadian rhythm disorders, which also include ACDs and ASPDs, will be reviewed briefly below, although there are others. ASPD therapy has rarely been studied by itself. According to personal communication, the chronobiotic melatonin has been used successfully. Recently, however, S. Campbell and M. Lovato investigated the effectiveness of melatonin, bright light and melatonin compared to the association of melatonin-bright light. However, even more complex are chronotherapy schedules: the most effective is complete sleep deprivation until the desired late bedtime and possibly 12 h of wake time, after which sleep re-enters, which has not yet been documented. All chronotherapy schedules seem to be effective if one wants to go to bed earlier rather than later within a few hours. For longer endogenous periods, light therapy alone appears to be more effective.

Till date, it is unclear to what extent environmental factors shape the onset and course of ASPD. First of all, it is very well possible that without an extreme influence it is impossible to become an evening-type. On the other hand, yet we do not know whether enforced early chronotypes automatically lead to an ASPD or if the unaffected ones escape into more common "eveningness" of the majority. In a first step towards understanding the disorder, we gathered reports from patients about possible triggering events occurring before the onset of the disorder. The information was collected through a self-designed questionnaire with a set of very concrete questions and additional empty fields. Fifty-two patients (14 men; 38 women) with ASPD were interviewed either personally or by e-mail. Forty different trigger events were reported, mainly a succession of two negative life events.

# 7. Diagnosis of Advanced Sleep Phase Disorder

Sleep Studies Sleep studies can aid in diagnosis. Multiple sleep latency tests (MSLT) should then be performed. The MSLT is useful if the patients are able to remain awake long enough for the assessment to be given. A MSLT should be performed on a representative evening and then at 7:00 p.m. PSG should be performed if nocturnal polysomnography is indicated. PSG/MSLT can be scheduled as early as 5:30 a.m. PSG can be performed after 5 hours of sleep in advance ASPD if hypersomnia is a concern. Treatment response to bright light therapy should guide therapy with patients who sleep during the afternoon. The treatment efficacy of morning or no bright light therapy in these patients is unknown.

Clinical Assessment Patients present with a consistent complaint of early evening falling asleep and pre-dawn awakening. The average age of onset is in the early fifties. They do not have difficulty consolidating sleep or staying awake during the day. Patients may mildly report difficulty with concentration and memory in the early evening. They may take short prophylactic early evening naps on a regular basis and awaken refreshed. There may be a family or personal history of other circadian rhythm sleep disorders. There may be a personal or family history of depression. Patients are typically morning larks. In very advanced ASPD, some patients go to bed once it is dark but then sleep for several hours until they awaken at 1-2 a.m.

and are unable to return to sleep. These patients will take naps during the afternoon.

Diagnosing Advanced Sleep Phase Disorder (ASPD) There is no gold standard test to diagnose advanced sleep phase disorder (ASPD). A clinical assessment and sleep studies can help medical professionals determine if this circadian rhythm disorder is present. The following procedures can help with diagnosis.

## 7.1. Clinical Assessment

Lately, some efforts have been made to harmonize criteria and guidelines for clinical and research purposes in circadian sleep-wake disorders, including ASPD, and there are two groups with initiatives of international impact. The research diagnostic criteria for advanced sleep phase disorder (ASPD) usually include the following: (1) Ages range from ~60 years to 80 years, occurring in 50% of cases, predominantly women, followed by men (28%); (2) A typical complaint is falling asleep or difficulty staying awake in the evening; (3) At least a 1-hour difference in sleep schedule along with criteria for circadian disorder or 1 to 3 pre-sleep issue signs and symptoms; and (4) The absence of prolonged evening bright light exposure in the evening with a possible decrease in cumulative lifetime photic exposure. Prospective diagnostics include symptoms ongoing since childhood or early adolescence, as well as symptoms not having occurred in the 3 months before examination or being in any other underlying sleep disorder such as sleep-related breathing or periodic limb movement disorder.

Differential diagnostic criteria for DSPD and ASPD from other sleep-wake disorders are lacking, and the assessment of these and other circadian sleep disorders in a clinical setting is challenging. Some differential clinical features of adult DSPD and ASPD cases were observed. DSPD cases tend to be more frequent in women ranging from adolescents to adults and in adulthood. In addition, DSPD cases were more symptomatic with the highest scores of daytime sleepiness, poorer sleep quality, and worst emotional experience. There are limited observations on the clinical assessment of ASPD. However, ASPD is, in general, a rare condition affecting elderly women with sensory impairment such as visual and/or hearing impairment, which can both account for the increasing prevalence trend and the phase advance for the treatment required in the diagnosis.

## 7.2. Sleep Studies

The usefulness of performing PSG to assess the pattern of an individual who presents for a dysregulation of their normal sleep-wake schedule is not of value. PSG should be considered in individuals meeting criteria for a diagnosis of ASWD where it is important to assess the presence or absence of other underlying sleep disorders to inform on what treatment is the best for the individual. Considering the sleep history, rather than PSG results, would be important when making a diagnosis of ASWD. PSG is more costly than an actigraphic assessment, it requires a trained technologist to attach the EOG and follow-up technical support which is not readily available. PSG is sorely limited as an outpatient assessment, requiring the participant to attend for a minimum of one overnight assessment in most cases since current-day wearables which enable home recordings are not clinically validated for multiple nights of use. PSG is an unnatural protocol for many and has technology that record brain wave EEG, ocular muscle activity via sEMG, and body muscle activity indicated by chin EMG. EEG uses a computer algorithm to record the electrical activity of the brain including the brain waves. The electrical activity of muscles is visualized by another device known as EMG. Ocular movements are detected through a device called EOG. Just prior to REM sleep, the body typically loses muscle tone. In subjects with PSG documentation of the above, all showed a significant shortening of sleep latency as a result of PSD.

A 14-day sleep diary, also known as a sleep-wake log, should be complemented by an actigraphy to confirm and quantify the advance of sleep timing. The assessment is conducted in ideal sleep environments: for sleep efficiency and Cape's values in advanced chronotypes, the availability of daytime sleeping protocols is recommended just as during the ESS. In case of suspected ASD, if other potential differential diagnoses have not yet been excluded, nighttime polysomnography (PSG) must be performed on a single night in order to exclude disorders including insomnia, narcolepsy, increased % of REM sleep or Periodic Limb Movements in Sleep. The advanced phase of the sleep-wake cycle can be assessed by protocols such as multiple sleep latency tests or polysomnographic cycles during the day to assess the phase angle between the melatonin onset and mid-sleep time, though no specific protocol is suggested in the ICCRD for research and/or diagnostic purposes at the time being. Actigraphy devices may or may not have the ability to measure other parameters including the intensity or duration of light exposure, and include an alarm to signal the subject to begin preparing for bed. Exact details of the actigraphy device used and the parameters included should be reported. Currently, there are several actigraphy devices that are approved by the US FDA, commercially available, but without published end of market applications that measure activity (motor activity or gross motor movements) or sleep/wake patterns.

# 8. Treatment Options

Compared to the rest of other pharmacological interventions, melatonin application may be of prime importance, as is its potent endogenous role, increasing in the evening for the induction of sleep, reducing in the morning for the gradual awakening and mobilization, and proven efficacy as an aid in facilitating the circadian system entrainment. As for the symptomatic patients with advanced sleep-wake syndrome, repeated administration of exogenous melatonin could be necessary for complaints improvement, and the evidence of its effective long-term compliance justifies the case-by-case judicious application of slow-release melatonin. Affordability and safety of the low dose-rate melatonin administration led this therapeutic option to be reported highly valuable by a non-anecdotal clinical community. The misalignment of the sleep-wake rhythm with the consecutive chronophysiological changes throughout the day leads to variable intensity of sleep inertia, the use of hypnotics possibly more harmful than beneficial. However, the early morning light therapy implemented in cases where critical early morning engagement is faced may be highly valuable in advancing sleep timing. Overall, the prognosis of the ASPD condition varies across the lifespan, but slow phase changes of the circadian system provide a moderate level of optimism for the ASPD individuals ready to sustain the scheduled time corrections in parallel to the clinical work of the managing psychiatrist.

Several pharmacological and non-pharmacological approaches are proven as valid treatment options for ASPD, although to date, there has been only one therapeutic agent, Hetlioz, registered for the treatment of ASPD. Among the non-pharmacological therapies, light therapy, chronotherapy, and social rhythm therapies gained considerable attention. Light therapy, often delivered by the means of the advance of sleep schedule shifted in line with the typical timing (20s/waking time phase) of melatonin and/or cortisol production coupled with the bright light exposure, has demonstrated high clinical efficacy for the system entrainment, in particular in the phase of evening types sleep-wake syndrome. However, also chronotherapy, administered at the timing of both melatonin and cortisol peak, led to promising results. Social rhythm therapy, focused on the wake-time regularity and the reduction of social role transitions among the working and school-age population, emphasizes the importance of the circadian system hygiene.

## 8.1. Non-Pharmacological Treatments

An additional non-pharmacological intervention for ASPD is the manipulation of the sleep-wake schedules. This treatment option includes advancing the bedtime and morning awakening using a chronotherapy approach. Individual factors should be considered when using this therapy such as the diurnal types, lifestyle, and available time. Providing psychoeducation was shown to increase circadian knowledge, sleep hygiene, subjective sleep quality, sleep time, and decreased sleep inertia. Relaxation therapies can reduce anxiety, and behavioral treatment and sleep hygiene were found to increase sleep duration in adults. Together with stress management, this therapy can reduce sleep disorders. Combination treatments combining non-pharmacological and pharmacological therapies have been suggested. These combination treatments can target the evening symptoms of ASPD and reduce exposure to hypnotic drugs in adults. Combination therapies are also of importance when treating treatment-resistant patients when using chronotherapy for ASPD. This may improve compliance and with the time of initiation of melatonin which should be started in the early morning. Combination therapies, focusing on sleep time, should also be initiated when using bright therapy as it exposes the eye area to a high dose of light which may reduce light perception. A chronopharmacology study should also consider the timing of providing bright light therapy and melatonin in addition to the regular bright light therapy or melatonin for people with ASPD symptoms in the evening. This can be investigated by comparing intervention versus placebo on changes in ASPD symptoms. 8.3. Limitations with Non-Pharmacological Treatments There is limited evidence on the effects of only using non-pharmacological approaches for ASPD. Psychoeducation has been shown to be one way that could be included in the treatment of ASPD. The treatment of ASPD when only focusing on non-pharmacological or combination therapy is a step in treatment. Sleep-wake therapies on the whole are not part of the American Academy of Sleep Medicine clinical guidelines, and adults with ASPD may have energy and mealtimes that are dysregulated which can affect metabolism. There is evidence to suggest that nutritional and exercise therapies in other disorders such as depression and anxiety can help with improvement in mood and functionality. A combined therapy approach using both chronotherapy and lifestyle deregulation—sleep-wake or mealtime—can have an effect on longer sleep duration independent of diagnosis. There are complications with lifestyle therapy including the difficulty of applying this treatment in those who are overweight, depressed, and cues with circadian function such as light exposure.

Non-pharmacological treatments. Several non-pharmacological interventions are available targeting the evening symptoms of ASPD, mostly based on behavior and lifestyle changes, including modulating light exposure, sleep-wake schedules, and sleep promotion modalities. The main evidence-based tools for regulating the circadian system are bright light therapy and scheduled behaviors. While bright light therapy is applied in the morning to delay sleep phase in people suffering from delayed sleep phase syndrome (DSPS) or be effective in the evening for advancing the circadian phase, it is not recommended for those with ASPD. Thus, we recommend evening dim light therapy. Similarly, scheduled behaviors are used to correct delayed circadian phase and are not relevant for the ASPD population who suffer from an evening shifted phase. Scheduled behaviors can be used to promote sleep and increase sleep continuity. Scheduled behaviors include sleep hygiene, bedtime restriction, stimulus control, and relaxation techniques (mindfulness or progressive muscle relaxation) which are considered to be effective for delayed sleep timing or insomnia. Increased physical activity is also recommended to promote daytime wakefulness.

## 8.2. Pharmacological Treatments

Bright light: Bright light in the evening has been shown to delay the phase of the body clock for individuals in the late-evening population. Pharmacologically, PDU was trialed by an Australian university hospital as a safe melatonin receptor 1,2 and 2/3 agonist. However, it was found in preliminary results to be ineffective in shifting the body clock, and hence people are no longer advised to take this medication. It is believed that ramelteon, an approved circadian rhythm treatment in the United States and marketed as Rozerem, may be an effective treatment for ASPD. Melatonin's derivative, agomelatine, acts as a melatonin receptor 1 and 2 agonist and has been reported in at least one case to be an effective treatment in ASPD.

Melatonin: Melatonin is the hormone that is typically released in response to darkness. It is the principal psychoactive chemical in the brain to signal that it is night. Melatonin's release advances the body temperature and begins to make the body feel sleepy, leading to a drop in the body clock's alertness. Melatonin needs to be taken several hours before intentional bedtime to serve as an advance shade signal. In general, most people who advance their sleep cycle more than 2 hours weekly are instructed to take melatonin 3 to 6 hours before bedtime.

A moderate number of pharmacological treatments showing promise for ASPD have been identified. These treatments largely target the circadian rhythm. The following is an overview of the medications that have been used to address ASPD; some of these medications are considered off-label treatment in Australia for ASPD.

Pharmacological treatments for ASPD

# 9. Lifestyle Modifications

(2) Overcoming the real issue of life modification: The majority of people with ASPD already have an irregular lifestyle and have difficulty finding work, attending for training, and carrying out activities committed to a schedule. A strict lifestyle would require significant effort and would have to be maintained for the rest of one's life. The person himself/herself and one's family should be conscious of the fact that these corrections are long-lasting and a lack of commitment to them may imply new risk conditions. Moreover, the person should be motivated and interested in keeping to a new timetable, being aware that maintaining it may produce a gradual improvement, reduce the risk of physical and mental illness such as cognitive impairment. If there is no interest and will to make any changes, clearly, a new timetable has little chance of being successful long term.

(3) Physical Activity: Regular physical activity is recommended as a good form of lifestyle management with benefits that go beyond improving sleep, including reducing symptoms of depression and anxiety which are also associated with sleep disorders. In the case of inappropriate lifestyle factors and lack of remission of symptoms, the combination of ET with light therapy could be considered to increase the beneficial effects on the sleep-wake cycle of people affected by ASPD. To date, this combined therapeutic approach has not yet been the

subject of any study or case report mentioned in the scientific literature.

(2) Modifying the sleep environment: In addition to light and dark exposure management, a comfortable sleep environment is also important as excessive noise and increased illumination or separate illumination of one partner could disturb sleep. Temporarily or for the more "stubborn" cases, in case of a more severe form of the disease, sleeping in a room separate from the rest of the family could be taken into consideration.

(1) Exposure to light and dark: Increased light exposure, especially in the morning, and decreased exposure before bedtime may be beneficial in the treatment of ASPD and may entrain the body clock to the correct circadian time (Class IIb; Level C).

The primary and most established recommendations for the management of ASPD involve behavioral or environmental factors that can be adopted on a daily basis. Adaptation to a schedule that allows habitually later bedtimes can benefit from a number of changes in this regard and the most common lifestyle guidelines suggested to people with ASPD are presented below.

## 10. Coping Strategies and Support

All participants revealed upsides and downsides to their advanced rhythms. As well as losing early evening energy, most lamented a loss of "contemplative" time alone. Some missed being with others and having company. Almost all complained of having to put up with the inconvenience of needing extra time in the morning to get through the AMS functions. But they did constantly try to find ways of adapting to the timing of their bodies, scheduling activities in the morning, lighting, eating, drinking, having time alone in the dark, meditating, etc. to make the best and worst of their evening and morning rhythms. Nobody articulated with their partners any conflicting tensions between how each lived or indicated any external support outside of the family that they were obtaining. They just got on with it on their own and in their own space.

The diagnosis of ASPD requires symptoms to have been present for at least three months. This means people diagnosed with ASPD have been living that way for quite some time before they enter assessment or treatment. This section focuses on how adults diagnosed with the condition come to understand it, what strategies they might use to get by, and how friends and family might help.

## 11. Research and Future Directions

ASP42_AD_AT_ASD is recognized by advanced research with regards to the characterization of patients undergoing MPS and ASPD by clinical and polysomnographical examinations. Research on ASPD is still being directed towards the fragmentation of the epidemiological, risk factors, biological, and comorbidity of PSD that have the current potential to reduce a great deal of the mysteries of PSD in general and ASPD in particular. The lack of research results also means that we are unable to obtain any clear conclusions on which conflict models should be presented. Hopefully, future mysteries will be resolved and detailed protocol attempts will be elaborated in order to aid this recent discovery.

Conclusions drawn from studies investigating the clinical profiles of patients with ASPD continue to be limited by cohort sample sizes (Table 1). Furthermore, most studies published on the topic used a retrospective design, limiting the generalizability of the findings. Few prospective, longitudinal studies have been completed. The database-wide observational studies were based on the questionnaires completed by the respondents and thus pulled from more accurate methodological approaches (e.g., MRI). Besides, self-report questionnaires are less objective in research investigating psychiatric disorders [62,63]. Future research should move away from retrospective chart analysis towards long-term, active methods such as inpatient or in-home actigraphy measurements. Current advances in bedside polysomnography provide quantitative methods to study the intracranial sleep-wake circuits of ASPD patients, including the timing of melatonin, body temperature, cortisol (basal and stress hormone), the ascending reticular activation system, narcolepsy antibodies, and orexin molecules. Each of these examinations is ready for planning in prospective, sleep-wake research.

# Advanced Sleep Phase Disorder: Causes, Symptoms, and Treatment Options

# 1. Introduction to Advanced Sleep Phase Disorder

Research into understanding ASPD has been protractedly meager due to a paucity of interest and the mistaken notion that ASPD itself is benign and does not warrant treatment. Plus, melatonin, the hormone that drives the propensity to sleep, is naturally secreted in a circadian time frame and not at artificially advanced times in the ASPD patient, as is witnessed in those individuals who find themselves compelled to sleep excessively advanced times. A general consensus was not arrived at until the last decade that ASPD is indeed an illness that requires treatment, and from there, how to manage and rectify such a proclivity to sleep.

Advanced Sleep Phase Disorder (ASPD) is characterized by the ability and sometimes the compulsion to sleep early at night, e.g. 6-9 PM, and waking as a consequence very early in the morning, e.g. 2-5 AM. This early morning waking does not arise from the person being dehydrated or any other physiological cause and is what differentiates ASPD from Early Morning Awakening Insomnia. When left to sleep in a more natural manner without a fixed routine, a person can be expected to sleep their fill of 7-9 hours, with no early waking. Hence, the symptoms and behaviors of the ASPD patient invariably align with the time they fall asleep and wake, and do not endorse the nighttime symptoms of secondary and primary insomnias.

Advanced Sleep Phase Disorder (ASPD) explained.

## 1.1. Definition and Overview

This neuroscience news article will provide an extensive look at Advanced Sleep Phase Disorder (ASPD), discussing the condition's root causes, the biological underpinnings, diagnosis options, how the disorder can impair a patient's quality of life, and potential treatment options. Advanced Sleep Phase Disorder (ASPD) can be difficult to contend with, as it does not necessarily produce insomnia, hypersomnia, or sleep continuity disturbances; however, the earlier bedtime poses potential difficulties for those living with the disorder. Within this node, we address some frequently asked questions about the disorder, including potential causes, information about ASPD's biological underpinnings, how the disorder can be diagnosed, potential therapies, and associated quality of life issues.

Advanced Sleep Phase Disorder is categorized under circadian rhythm sleep disorders, which are characterized by disruptions in a person's circadian rhythm. A circadian rhythm refers to physical, mental, and behavioral changes that follow a 24-hour cycle. These biological processes are primarily influenced by environmental cues, and they are often referred to as a person's internal body clock. Circadian rhythm sleep disorders can manifest from various triggers, including shift work, time zone changes, lifestyle changes, work schedules, and other issues that can compromise the normal functioning of the circadian clock. Advanced Sleep Phase Disorder (ASPD) is classified as a sleep-wake circadian rhythm sleep disorder in the fifth edition of the Diagnostic and Statistical Manual of Mental Disorders (DSM-V).

## 2. Understanding Circadian Rhythms

Advanced Sleep Phase Disorder (ASPD), or circadian rhythm sleep disorder, is a sleep disorder characterized by changes in gene structure or other factors that drive it. A chronotype is a person's natural rhythm, analogous to early risers (morning) and night owls (evening). Since childhood or adolescence, people who are morning or evening types have noticed that their patterns are considerably more rigid than usual. ASPD, except for the regular 7-8 hours of sleep, has more serious effects than simple morning orientation. According to one scenario, ASPD patients cannot remain awake for a reasonable amount of time after awakened (earlier). Falling asleep before the bedtime of regular society (usually 10-11 pm) is problematic. Despite remaining in bed for hours, showing constant adaptation to extraordinary stress throughout their lives has little effect on their Standard Time of Awakening performance.

Each person's body operates on a 24-hour cycle, which is formalized as their "circadian rhythm". A natural schedule called a circadian rhythm regulates several physical, emotional, and behavioral patterns, including the sleep-wake cycle. The circadian rhythm of a person is influenced by numerous things, including how recently they were awake, whether or not their body has a normal sleep pattern, the consistency of their sleep, their exposure to light, and a hormone in their brain. It's hard to adjust disrupted circadian rhythms because so many body functions are involved. Irregular sleep patterns may result from changes in body rhythms. The human body can produce various sleep disturbances as a result of the body clock's disturbance.

## 2.1. What is a Circadian Rhythm?

Body temperature, hormone precursors, levels of hormones, and neurotransmitters are also affected by our circadian rhythm. As a result, healthy physiology of the heart, gastrointestinal system, liver, and other systems are affected. This variation can result in many symptoms such as changes in alertness or levels of cognitive functioning, mood, energy, and stamina. The rhythms of various systems reach a peak during the biological prime time, which produces a person's utmost physical and energy strength, which then decreases through the biological low. In implicitly relating to humans, the regulation of time is influenced by our own internal clocks that are kept in rhythm with light, hormones, and the environment around us.

Our body has a 24-hour cycle referred to as a circadian rhythm. Each individual's biological clock aligns to a slightly different schedule. Everyone experiences a time period that they are the most awake and alert known as the biological prime time or chronotype, and a time of decreased alertness known as the biological low or the sleep phase. These rhythms are affected by various stimuli and habits in our daily lives. Some of these influencing factors include exposure to light or darkness, physical activity, and food intake. Approximately every 24.2 hours our biological rhythms require us to sleep, relax, and rest so that they are able to re-adjust. While doing this, the time in which sleep is needed can fluctuate or be extended, and the rhythms are regulated and restarted.

# 3. Causes of Advanced Sleep Phase Disorder

The disorder has been linked to several genes, including: PSVT1, a protein-coding gene that may provide the body's circadian rhythm signals. In 2015, Lois Krahn, a out of Mayo Clinic, and David Christensen, first author out of University of Minnesota Duley Center, further linked ASPD to the gene PER3 which also affects an individual's typical wake up time. According to the research, people with one or both of PER3's genetic variants have an average circadian wake-up time of 6:07 a.m., regardless of their work schedules. Variants of PER3 are associated with shorter and longer sleep times as well, so it can be the source of a different sleep disorder. All of these factors get mixed together and can result in an ASPD diagnosis. The onset of ASPD is typically benign, meaning that symptoms are relatively mild and do not cause significant lifestyle changes. Symptom severity may progressively worsen with age, with more moderate to severe forms of the disorder presenting later in life.

The exact origins of advanced sleep phase disorder remain a matter of scientific study. As of now, it's estimated that roughly four percent of the adult population in the United States have been diagnosed with this sleep disorder, but it's likely that many more are living with this condition without a proper diagnosis. This condition can significantly impact an individual's quality of life and is a common diagnosis in sleep medicine practices. Since there is no clear way to weed out those without ASPD, the four percent figure likely includes people who are living with rare sleep conditions that could be contributing to their chronotype. There are known factors to contribute to ASPD. It's believed that in some individuals, the onset of sleep lays naturally outside the range of typical sleep patterns. Ongoing genetic studies are attempting to identify the genes underlying this difference.

## 3.1. Genetic Factors

The evidence presented in the last section underlines that ASPD is not the result of a regular sleep pattern after two cycles of 24 h, but a circadian phase disorder. Heritability of the circadian period length has been suggested in twin studies. In a 1999 study, an inheritable contributor to a shorter free-running circadian rhythm (phase angle between melatonin onset and wake-up time) was found in a set of 49 blind individuals. However, this has not been observed in sighted patients with hereditary ASPD. Possibly, such heritability has not yet emerged because current research is focusing on one of the most extreme ends of the circadian rhythm spectrum. It might also be possible that the very small group of 21 ASPD patients studied so far lacks the power to observe this effect. Further genetic research is however necessary and could perhaps be more rewarding, as the precise genetic modulation might lie downstream in the many processes in which the core clock plays a regulatory role in the body. The genetic basis of this condition is still largely undetermined. The autosomal-dominant inheritance pattern in some families at least supports the notion that genetic factors contribute to the development of ASPD.

Circadian rhythms are regulated by an internal time-keeping system, where genetic factors are thought to be important. In mammals, the central clock resides in the suprachiasmatic nucleus (SCN) of the hypothalamus and acts as a master pacemaker, controlling peripheral oscillators in other organ systems through autonomic and endocrine outputs. The current model of the basic molecular mechanism underlying the circadian clock is a transcriptional auto-regulatory feedback network formed by several core clock genes and their protein products. Briefly, CLOCK (circadian locomotor output cycles kaput) and BMAL1 (brain, muscle, aryl hydrocarbon receptor nuclear translocator like) proteins heterodimerize and bind to the E-box elements of clock genes, period (PER1, PER2, and PER3) and cryptochrome (CRY1 and CRY2), and repress their transcription. The CLOCK:BMAL1:PER:CRY transcriptional repression loop constitutes not only the core feedback loop of the molecular oscillator but is also thought to be the site of the master regulatory action of the circadian clock. The CLOCK:BMAL1 complex also regulates the transcription of other clock-controlled genes (CCGs) through D-box elements in their promoters. The resultant protein products control downstream processes.

# 4. Symptoms and Diagnosis

Preferably, the signs and symptoms of ASPD are directly related to the circadian phase in question, but they commonly present in opposition to the circadian phase that it coincides with. Preliminary diagnoses for ASPD are reached through clinical presentations that demonstrate the symptoms of the disorder, which include having a particular circadian lifestyle that is advanced relative to normal life. The most often recognized clinical cases of ASPD without a family history are virtual cases in treatment-seeking individuals. That is because these are the people who develop an alarm phase of somewhat permanent early awakening, and when there is no reading of the initial delayed sleep phase, the disorder fits the description of having begun in late adolescence or adulthood. One case was identified in a 3-year-old boy who had delayed sleep onset and some capacity to sleep later given the opportunity.

The key symptoms of ASPD are an early awakening time and an inability to sleep later than average, followed by a gradual decline in energy and alertness as the day goes on, which can result in serious problems if formal obligations require them to stay awake for longer. A definitive diagnosis for ASPD is usually made with a sleep diary, with polysomnography used to rule out other sleep disorders. In everyday life, it can be diagnosed with Actigraphs, which are a type of watch that individuals wear and monitor their sleep schedules. While delayed sleep phase preference

(DSPP) does exist, it operates on a different timeframe than that of ASPD; it has a clock that is an hour or so behind, keeping an otherwise typical day-night cycle in place. The signs and symptoms of ASPD, as well as the appearance of the circadian rhythm, are in direct contrast to those of DSPP, demonstrating everything.

## 4.1. Common Symptoms

All individuals with only one exception, noted within our office, appeared to be more efficient during the morning hours. The one exception was a partner of a retired CEO who was not required to go to work until noon or later and could accomplish many tasks until that time. However, when the individual was younger and had to get ready for school, she could barely function. It is important to emphasize that at any age, delays in sleep-wake cycles, most commonly delayed sleep phase disorder, can exhibit the extreme manifestation of ASPD. Sleep diaries and actigraphy can be helpful in diagnosis, as well as assisting in developing an appropriate entrainment plan. Treatment to realign sleep/wake cycles for those who want to sleep more than 3 hours over and above their habitual sleep period are most successful if the treatment starts on a weekend or at the start of a vacation.

The most common symptoms of ASPD include early awakenings, which in its most extreme presentation can happen as early as 1 or 2 a.m. However, there can be individuals who have a more moderate presentation, waking up between 3 to 6 a.m. ASF individuals tend to be "morning people" and therefore tend to be more alert and function more effectively during the morning hours. Finally, people with ASPD will go to bed early, generally between 6 p.m. to 9 p.m., but this time can be influenced by sociocultural influences, particularly as one gets older. The condition can affect all age groups, but a propensity for inheritance is suspected. ASPD occurs more commonly in older individuals and is thought to be more prevalent in women than men.

# 5. Treatment Options

The CPAP device is the most categorically indicated treatment for moderate to severe OSA. In the available review of multiple studies of melatonin in delayed sleep phase and other circadian rhythm problems, mild benefits such as enhanced sleep and daytime general well-being have been suggested. Agomelatine regularizes the circadian body rhythm and reduces depressive symptoms. Likewise, it's anything more to fall asleep or stay asleep. If you've tried everything else and can't find the precise moment, we generally change the dose, the amount, and the phenotype of the patient. PSG must be retuned to determine the most delayed sleep episode and define the new awakening episode and participate in the strict schedule of the new sleep period for about three weeks. Risperidone: not just to fall asleep or stay asleep. You can resleep even after getting up the bulk of our plan, and the like. The schedule must be followed severely for about three weeks.

The goal of any treatment strategy for advanced sleep phase disorder is to establish a stable schedule and a suitable rhythm. The proper hour of going to bed must be shifted late, and it should be consistent with when sleep occurs and finishing it on the rhythm. This approach favors a few hours of wear. Most medications for treating advanced sleep phase disorder have been effective in delivering only short-term gains and with a measure of side effects.

## 5.1. Medications

Melatonin agonists may be used, though study data is scarce on effects in ASPD. Agonists for the melatonin 1 (MT1) and melatonin 2 (MT2) receptor are classified as ramelteon, agomelatine, and tasimelteon. Ramelteon is licensed in the USA for primary insomnia for up to 35 days, and for ASPS, there are no head-to-head RCTs with melatonin or placebo. Agomelatine spent some time in the spotlight because of a supposedly lower negative effect on sleep architecture and the likelihood of fewer addiction rates. In head-to-head studies, ramelteon seems as beneficial as agomelatine, but the latter is also not approved for long-term use. Ramelteon was awarded FDA license for children and adolescents in 2020 with 2 RCTs stating effectiveness. Dosage for ASPS: 1.5-8mg.

Melatonin is a natural hormone that our bodies produce and plays a main role in the sleep-wake cycle. Melatonin supplements are widely and safely used in the treatment of sleep disorders, and this may include the use of melatonin as an adjunct treatment for circadian rhythm sleep disorders, especially in combination with light therapy. Retrospective chart reviews and some controlled studies have reported melatonin benefits in ASPS, especially when combined with bright light therapy. It can also be used by itself in patients with no access to bright light therapy. Reported dosages range from 0.5 to 12mg taken 4-5 hours before sleep. Although melatonin itself may cause sleepiness, "rebound" alerting effects may occur as levels decline and have been reported in some studies. There was also concern about chronic administration of large doses, such as momentary strong sedative effect (activation after) and low dose long-term activation due to fewer receptors. It is available over the counter.

Commonly used medications

## 5.2. Light Therapy

There are speculations that light therapy can be effective for treating DSPD and ASPD. The one study that investigated treatment of ASPD with light therapy suggested an antidepressant effect with the treatment, as well as a suggestion that the treatment's onset is about 4 hours after the timing of the release of melatonin to the treatment. However, that study treated patients with ASPD with bright light (10,000 lux) from 10pm-2am and did not analyze circadian phase markers in the study. In short, light therapy theoretically could be effective for the treatment of ASPD, but to date there is no direct evidence that light therapy is an effective treatment. Similarly, in our opinion, there is definitely potential for diluting the selection of patients that meet criteria for ASPD in clinical trials of light therapy, and so one must keep these things in mind when evaluating whether light therapy is the correct treatment option for an ASPD patient. Brief exposure to light in the morning, 30-120 minutes after waking, is a recommended approach for treating DSPD with light. Future studies are necessary to determine the validity of light therapy for ASPD.

Light therapy: Light therapy is a non-pharmacological approach that helps treat a variety of sleep disorders, including circadian rhythm sleep disorders, major depressive disorder with a seasonal pattern, jet lag, and shift work disorder. Light therapy involves using light boxes, dawn simulators, and light glasses. Therapeutic light intensity should have a brightness of at least 2,500 lux. The time of administration of light can range from eight hours before to ten hours after the core body temperature minimum. However, for most individuals, treating during the first or second part of the biological night is most effective.